The Caregiver's Cliff Notes:

27 Things to Do When Your Parents Are Losing Their Independence

By Stella Nsong, RN, CMC, CDP, LTCP

Copyright © 2013 Stella Nsong.

ISBN 978-0-9881914-4-0

Author's Website

www.StellaNsong.com

The Caregiver's Cliff Notes:

27 Things to Do When Your Parents Are Losing Their Independence

"This carefully-crafted yet concise book is an excellent and very readable guide for finding one's way through the frightening landscape of assisting aging parents when they need more care than their children can provide. This book gives you an easy to understand plan, actionable steps and practical solutions that you can use right on the spot. It's a must read if you have an aging loved one." — ***Dr. Esther Hampton, Ph.D.***

.

"EXCELLENT, inspiring, informational read concerning the progressive process of aging and the complexity of Caregiving. A must for any baby boomer." — ***William C. Bailey, RN, Vice President, Distinguished Orthopedic Home Care***

Table of Contents

Introduction

My name is Stella Nsong. I am a nurse entrepreneur. I have been a nurse for over twenty years and a real entrepreneur for about fifteen years.

In my everyday life, I do not practice a lot of clinical nursing. What I practice every day is lamp lighting... my art of shedding the light that you can use to find your way in whatever situation life has placed you. Someone once told me that I am actually a "*laugh* lighter" because I have a loud laugh and one of those big, contagious smiles that can light up a third-world country.

Over the last twenty years, I have mastered the care of the elderly. I have learned and developed effective strategies to encourage older adults to do what they *should* be doing–and I have actually found the way to help them *enjoy* what they are supposed to be doing. I have helped hundreds of families go through care, surgeries, rehabilitation, hospice care, death and dying.

> **This little book will encourage you, help you stay on top of your caregiving situation, and help you to keep things in perspective.**

Along with my staff and clients, we have rejoiced, laughed and cried through all sorts of caregiving situations. I have learned quite a few lessons that I share with you in these pages. I hope to bring joy to your heart, a smile even when you are tired and exhausted, and to be a lamp of light to help you find your way or to ignite the joy and hope that you need to carry out your caregiving responsibilities.

This little book will encourage you, help you stay on top of your caregiving situation, and help you to keep things in perspective. Enjoy the quotes, laugh really loud when you can, and remember that sometimes the strongest thing you can do is to ask for help.

When you read some of these stories, you will realize that you are not alone. And if you feel up to it, by all means, get up and dance as if no one is looking. Now, sit, clear your head, relax, and let's journey together and remember two things:

1. When things go wrong, don't go with them.

2. In caregiving, love is not enough.

Mary Claire

How to Get the Best Use out of this Book

My intent for this book is to give you a quick, useful reference, packed with action steps that you can use right now to get help quickly before you lose your mind. If it feels like it is too late and you are already losing your mind, then my hope is to help you find the assistance you need so that you can regain control of the situation.

Each chapter begins with a powerful quote and ends with a powerful caregiving tip and a small section for your notes. The quotes will help you to keep things in perspective. The tips will help you get organized if you choose to explore the tips. Place a check mark in the box as you complete each of them and by the time you get to the end of the book and all your check marks are in place, you will be very much in control of your Caregiving situation. I have written quite a few caregiving stories as well. All of them are true and happened in my practice. I tell you true stories to help you relate, to help you realize that you are not alone, to motivate you to get your plan together, and to help you keep sane.

Chapter 9 has three important guides that will help you find the best in-home medical and non-medical agency or assisted living community for your given situation.

Chapter 10 is a long term care planning survey which will help you know what to do next and which kind of help you really need. The care planning survey will also help you to keep guilt in check because you will be able to determine the long term care wishes of your parents. The results of the survey will guide you towards their preferences for their future long term care setting.

By the time you get to the end of the book, you will have regained control of the situation. You will be able to help your parents feel as independent as possible, while getting more life out of days than days out of life. This little book is sure to vaporize and float the caregiving stress right out of your life.

CHAPTER 1

Caregiving Shop Talk:

Big complex words simplified.

This chapter introduces you to the language that you will hear when discussing your parents' health issues with the eldercare professionals. Those big and complex expressions are simplified so that you will know what the heck they are really talking about.

Understanding the Language of Eldercare.

The first time you consider care for an elder family member, you will hear all sorts of new and different words. Eldercare has its own language, including terms that involve legal, financial and insurance documents. This brief glossary will help you know what everyone's talking about.

Long Term Care

When people hear the term "long term care," most automatically think of nursing homes. Long term care really means the place where a senior will spend most of the last days of his or her life. It is the place where they will stay as they age—be it long term care in their own home, the home of family or friends, a retirement community, an independent living complex, adult day care, an assisted living facility, or a nursing home.

Activities of Daily Living (ADL)

A critical part of independent living is the ability to complete basic functions of daily living. Going to the bathroom, taking a shower, dressing, combing your hair, brushing your teeth and shaving are what are collectively known as Activities of Daily Living. If there is a problem with any of these activities, there is a problem staying independent.

Instrumental Activities of Daily Living (IADL)

Using the telephone, writing a letter, driving a car, shopping, cooking, cleaning, paying bills and managing medications are collectively known as Instrumental Activities of Daily Living. Although these functions are essential to daily living, they are not critical in determining independent living because they can be resolved by involving other caregiving people like you and those that are substituting for you.

Durable General Power of Attorney

This legal document gives power to another person to make legal or financial decisions such as check writing, banking and tax preparation if you are unable to do so. These powers can be made narrow or broad. Be careful when using a form to assign power of attorney because some forms are not legally binding. It is best to have this document prepared by an attorney, signed and notarized.

Durable Power of Attorney for Health Care

This legal document gives power to another person to make medical decisions if you are unable to do so. It should be used along with a living will. Living wills are limited to life and death medical care. You can obtain the form for a power of attorney for health care from the state bar association. A durable power of attorney for health care must be signed and notarized to be considered legal in most states.

Advanced Directive

A legal document that allows a person to express wishes in advance to let medical professionals know what medical treatments are acceptable in the event of terminal illness or temporary incapacity. The living will directive supersedes the durable power of attorney for health care. Consult with a physician.

Conservatorship

This is created voluntarily at the request of a physically infirmed but competent adult to place his/her property or person under court supervised care.

Dementia

Simply means the loss of intellectual functions (such as memory deficit, poor judgment or confusion) that interfere with daily living. Many conditions cause or mimic dementia including brain tumors, depression, adverse drug interaction and nutritional deficiencies. A geriatric assessment can help to determine the cause of dementia and suggest treatment that can improve or even reverse behavior patterns.

Level of Care Assessment

A level of care assessment is a set of criteria developed by each state to determine if a person meets medical eligibility for institutional or community based care programs. A level of care assessment is usually conducted by a licensed professional such as a social worker or a nurse and it takes into consideration a person's medical, health and psychosocial needs. Each state tailors its own criteria so someone eligible for services in the state of Ohio may not be eligible in the state of Oklahoma.

Medicare

Medicare is a federal health insurance program for people age 65 and older and for certain disabled individuals. There is part A, B and D.

Medicare Part A

Medicare part A is hospital insurance which helps pay for care in a hospital and skilled nursing facility, home health care and hospice care.

Medicare Part B

Medicare part B is supplemental insurance. It pays for outpatient care medical services, doctor bills, home health care, lab fees, therapies and ambulance services. This part of Medicare is optional and has a monthly premium based on your income. If you do not want part B, you must decline it or else it will be automatically deducted from your social security check.

Medicare Part D

People with Medicare have the option of paying a monthly premium for outpatient prescription drug coverage. This prescription drug coverage is called Medicare Part D. Generally, you will pay out of pocket for monthly Part D premiums and also pay 100% of your drug cost until a certain deductible amount is reached. After reaching the deductible, you pay a percentage of your drug cost and the part D premium pays the rest until the total you and your plan spend on your drugs reaches $2800. Once you reach this limit, you have hit the coverage gap referred to as the "donut hole." You are now responsible for the full cost of your drugs until the total you have spent for your drugs reaches the yearly out-of-pocket spending limit of approximately $4550.00. The donut hole ranges from $2700 to $6153.73 based on the person and their Part D drug coverage.

CAREGIVER TIP:

The three most important documents you need to assume responsible caregiving of a loved one or to protect your wishes are: a **general durable power of attorney** (for financial and legal), a **living will** and a **durable power of attorney for health care**. Make sure all copies are signed and notarized. It is important to tell your doctor, executor, family members and close friends that you have these documents and exactly where they are located.

NOTES:

_____

_____

_____

_____

_____

_____

_____

_____

   Get signed, notarized legal documents in place.

CHAPTER 2

The Role of the Care Manager:
What to do if suddenly
everything has hit the fan...

This chapter introduces you to care management and the role that a care manager can play in your caregiving situation. A care manager is a social worker or a nurse who does assessments, care planning, care coordination and care management to make sure that the care that is provided is achieving its purpose towards safety, recovery and quality of life. Usually, there is a fee for this service. In times of crisis, especially in long distance caregiving, a care manager can save you a lot of time, energy and stress.

"Being out of control is one of the worst feelings

in the world, sometimes even worse than pain.

It is its own kind of pain"

– Danzae Pace

The Police, the Son, Mom, and her 88-Year-Old Boyfriend
...a True Story

"What is your emergency?" answered the 911 operator.

Neighbor reporting: "There is a half-naked lady wandering in her yard, and she can't seem to find her way back into the house."

Minutes afterwards, the police show up and confirm the situation. Inside the house, which is filthy, the police discover the wandering lady's 88-year-old boy friend—who is also very frail and ill, and unable to care for himself.

The police officer places a call to adult protective services. Right in the middle of their phone conversation, the lady's 60-something-year-old son pulls up in the driveway.

The son had moved into town two years ago to care for mom and her boyfriend. He was living in mom's boyfriend's home while providing care to them two to three times a day. The problem was the son was also very ill. As a matter of fact, because of his terminal diagnosis, the son could probably die before mom and boyfriend.

The son, with all his good intentions, had started working on power of attorney documents so he could manage mom and mom's boyfriend's affairs. Mom's boyfriend has no children and no close relatives but owns a nice house. The police officer makes a deal with the son to arrange for care right away, or else mom and her boyfriend will be sent to the hospital and then placed in a nursing home.

Ring, ring, ring – and that was my telephone ringing and their lawyer saying to me, "Please rescue my clients... do something today, or they will be placed in a nursing home!"

That is when I got involved. I started with round-the-clock care, mental health assessments, new medications, long term care planning, and lots and lots of complex caregiving issues.

Come to find out, the power of attorney documents the son had just worked on were no good, because mom and her boyfriend were recently diagnosed with dementia. There was not enough money to pay for care, so a reverse mortgage and cashing of the IRAs were in order.

Yet all of that had to be stopped because the son did not have authority to execute these decisions after all. He had waited too long to obtain the powers of attorney. And, because of the recent diagnosis of dementia, the power of attorney documents where no good.

Long story short, they all ended up in the nursing home against their wishes because there were no "good" documents in place, no long term care plans, no wills and no willing family members to help out. Mom's house and her boyfriend's house, all worth over $300,000 dollars, will end up in estate recovery while they live in the nursing home.

Action Plan:

When everything hits the fan, get a care manager right away. He or she will help sort through the complex situations and help get things under control very quickly. Here are:

The Top 10 Things Care Managers Can Help You With

1. Conduct a level of care assessment to identify caregiving problems and to recommend caregiving solutions.

2. Provide crisis intervention in the home, at a hospital and at a care facility.

3. Screen, match and arrange for in-home help or other caregiving services including assistance in hiring qualified caregivers at home.

4. Function as a liaison to families who are far away and even those who are close by for overseeing, coordinating and responding to family members in the event of a caregiving problem.

5. Facilitating the relocation of an older adult to and from a retirement community, assisted living facility or a nursing home.

6. Provide advocacy and eldercare education to families and other care team members.

7. Provide eldercare counseling and support.

8. Review financial, legal and medical issues and offer referrals to all appropriate medical and care specialists.

9. Provide financial, legal and medical review and assessments for the application of benefits including Veterans Administration Aid and Attendance benefits, long term care insurance and state medical waivers.

10. Help family members keep SANE and to find MEANING and JOY as they juggle responsibilities in all their caregiving roles.

Top 3 Places to Look when You Need a Care Manager Right Away

1. National Care Planning Council
   www.longtermcarelink.net

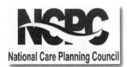

2. National Association of Professional Geriatric Care Managers
   www.caremanager.org

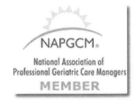

3. National Academy of Certified Care Managers
   www.NACCM.net

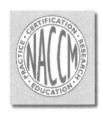

CAREGIVER TIP:

The body disposes of medications differently as a person ages. Sometimes older adults can experience emotional difficulties and behave strangely due to medication that they are taking. Make sure that your loved one uses only one pharmacy and that you know the names, dosages, possible side effects, what to do about missed doses and any special storage instructions of all their medications.

NOTES:

_____

_____

_____

_____

_____

_____

_____

_____

Organize medication information and pharmacy access.

CHAPTER 3

Balanced Caregiving:

How to manage a caregiving crisis when money is tight.

This chapter will give you a step-by-step plan for getting good care when your parents can't afford a certified geriatric care manager or when there is a caregiving crisis and no time to wait for a care manager to get back to you.

"That the birds of worry and care fly over your head, this you cannot change, but that they build nests in your hair, this you can prevent"

— Chinese Proverb

The Key to Balanced Caregiving

For a majority of Americans, eldercare has become a frustrating do-it-yourself process. This is because long term care services are complicated and provider contacts are fragmented throughout the community. Using professional services helps relieve stress, reduces conflict and saves time and money. Hiring professional advisers and providers to help with long term care is no different than using professionals to help with other complex issues such as car repairs, taxes and legal affairs.

In much the same way as a three-legged stool needs all three legs to be useful, the care giving approach needs at least *three key elements* in order to be successful with as little stress as possible. It needs

- ✓ **You**

- ✓ **Eldercare Professionals, and**

- ✓ **Government/Community Long Term Care Programs.**

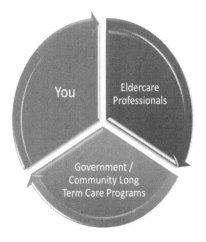

Three Key Elements of Balanced, Affordable Caregiving

Long Distance Caregiving: A True Story

Mary is a great neighbor. She looks out for her 83-year-old friend Bob, who lives next door in a small house with falling gutters, over-grown grass lawn, and a very cluttered driveway.

Bob has a son who lives on the west coast. The son has a young family, and a demanding job that requires extensive travel. He usually visits his dad about once every other year; however, he has not seen his dad in over three years due to work and the bad economy. He and his dad have discussed having power of attorney documents put in place several times in the past. The son relies heavily on Mary (the neighbor) for information about his dad.

Mary travels to visit her family over the weekend. On her return, she finds Bob sitting in his car in 93° heat, covered with bruises, very tired and probably dehydrated. A stubborn ex-marine, Bob refuses to go to the hospital for fear that they will keep him there, take away his license, and ask him to move into a nursing home. Apparently, Bob had been threatened with losing his independence in similar situations in the past.

His son cannot come from the west coast to be with him. Mary moves in with Bob to provide round-the-clock care, but because she works part time, Mary can only stay with Bob for about two days straight.

In the meantime, Bob has fallen twice since Mary moved in. The son, now worried sick about his dad's situation, wants to get dad some help right away. Bob tells his son he will think about the power of attorney document. The son has heard about VA benefits, and he thinks now it will be a good time to check into things.

Next thing you know, my phone was ringing – and here is how we handled the situation.

Action Steps to Identify Care Needs

Action Step #1: Determine the Safety Factors

First we answered the following **7 safety questions**:

1. Can dad safely ambulate in his home?

2. Is he eating and has he lost weight?

3. Is he taking his medications?

4. Does dad have the money for round-the-clock care?

5. Is dad being treated for an infection?

6. What is dad's monthly income with assets?

7. Is dad resistant to care?

Answer Key to the 7 Safety Questions – what the answers may mean and what you can do about them:

1. **If dad cannot safely ambulate**, you run the risk of a fall and a fracture which could mean the end of dad's ability to remain independent. A fall is a defining event in the life of an older adult. Fifty percent of older adults who fall and sustain a hip fracture will die within a year.

2. **If dad has lost weight**, there are more problems with his care. Dehydration usually goes with weight loss.

3. **If dad is not taking his medications**, he might need to be admitted to the hospital for a complete workup because non-compliance with medication can compound his health issues. If, for example, he should be taking blood thinners and he has not been, you have an emergency on your hands.

4. **Round-the-clock care** can range from $9.00 to $21 dollars an hour. If dad does not have this in his budget, the hospital is your next bet.

5. **If dad is being treated for an infection**, then his safety concerns will gradually subside. It may take up to 2 weeks for an older adult to respond to antibiotics after an infection. An infection could cause an older adult to fall or to have symptoms that look like dementia.

6. **If dad's monthly income and assets are not enough** for care management and round-the-clock care right now, consider sending dad to the hospital. There comes a time when not having a lot of money may not be a very bad thing. This is why Medicaid exists to help dad when his income is not enough.

7. **If dad is resistant to care** and you are far away, the Department of Job and Family Services is now your partner in care. There is hope – so here is what we did for Bob and his long distance caregiver son.

Action Step #2: Involve Professional Services

Here was Bob's situation:

> He was falling, covered in bruises, his memory was failing him, he had lost a lot of weight, had not been to the doctor in a long time, had no savings, monthly income was less than $2000, he lived in a rented house, is a veteran (but had not applied for benefits) and he was resistant to care.

We called the ambulance and sent Bob to the hospital. The hospital kept him for several days. When he became medically stable, they sent him for rehabilitation placement, and then placement into an assisted living facility under Medicaid, with a court-appointed guardian.

This was the best solution for Bob considering the situation. He thrived thereafter, made a lot of good friends and enjoyed his time with other guys his age who also served in the military.

Your Action Plan for Balanced Caregiving

- Identify and write down your needs as the caregiver in your situation.

- Call the eldercare locator number which is **1-800-677-1116**.

  The eldercare locator is a national toll free referral number funded by the Administration on Aging. You can call this number with questions and they will direct you to a specialist in your area who can help you.

- Call your local **Area Agency on Aging** for a free resources guide.

  There are approximately 655 area agencies on aging in every state and territory of this country. These agencies concentrate primarily on helping elderly people remain independent in the community, delaying the need for placement into a facility. These agencies also administer the family caregiver support program and coordinate Medicaid programs for home care and assisted living. Most of them have a resource guide that has a listing of all the providers you will need to make your 3-legged plan for balanced caregiving successful.

Eldercare Locator Number: 1-800-677-1116

CAREGIVER TIP:

Schedule a level of care assessment so that you know how much care is needed now versus what may be needed in the future so that you have enough information to develop a solid long term care plan. Through the elder care locator, you will be able to locate the nearest Area Agency on Aging. More often than not, these assessments are free.

NOTES:

_____

_____

_____

_____

_____

_____

_____

_____

Schedule a level of care assessment.

CHAPTER 4

How to Get Your Parents to Listen to You:
What to say and when to say it.

In this chapter, we will look at ways you can approach the topic of supportive living with your parents. By following these guidelines when expressing your concerns, your chances of being heard will be increased. Good advice can be great and it makes a difference who gives it.

*"The turning point in the process of growing up
is when you discover the core strength
within you that survives all hurt"*

— Max Lerner, The Unfinished Country, 1950

Action Plan for Getting Your Parents to Listen to You

The way you approach your parents about your concerns can have a tremendous impact on how receptive they are.

First, know your reason for raising your concerns. Here are a few questions to ask yourself.

1. Do you want to discuss an issue or do you want mom and dad to do what you think needs to be done?

2. Are you acting out of concern or out of self interest?

3. Do you want mom and dad to make a change because it will enhance their independence or because it will make you worry less?

4. Do your parents have specific challenges or have there been incidences that warrant change? Or, are you concerned simply because of their age?

Good advice can be great advice based on who it is coming from. Get the doctor to discuss issues like driving and the use of assistive devices such as canes and walkers.

Being told by a doctor that a person can no longer drive because of health reasons will be a more acceptable reason for not driving than for a relative saying, "You are no longer a good driver" or "You should sell your car."

> *"The way you approach your parents about your concerns can have a tremendous impact on how receptive they are."*

Another good way to handle the issue of driving is to have your parents go through the occupational therapy driving assessment. If they fail the driver's test, then the issue is resolved without you being the bad child that thinks that mom or dad is no longer a good driver. You will need a doctor's order for the insurance company to cover a portion of the cost. A good way to begin this discussion is at the doctor's office during an annual physical when vision has to be checked.

What to Say, and When to Say It

It is good to take action during moments of normal interaction *before* a situation becomes a crisis. For example:

When Susie saw her dad having trouble reaching for items in the upper kitchen cabinet, she said,

> "I see those cupboards are really high. I saw the neatest thing that can
> reach those high places. How about I get you one of them and we can try
> it. You tell me what to put on which shelf and we see how it works."

When you talk about the high cupboard being the problem rather than dad having a problem, you make dad feel in control and more receptive to your suggestion. Take responsibility for your concerns. Your parents will listen to you if you express your concerns in terms of your feelings rather than as though your parents have problems.

When you talk to your parents in 'I' statements, you communicate concern and caring. When you talk to them in "you" statements, your messages sound accusatory and dictatorial.

Instead of saying:

- "Dad, you are too old to be climbing a ladder and cleaning the gutters. You ought to hire someone to do it."

- "You are no longer safe on the road. You drive like a maniac."

- "Mom, your neighbors are complaining about how loud your TV is. The management may ask you to move out."

Try saying it this way:

- "Dad, I really worry when you are up on the ladder and no one is around. I am worried that you might fall and hurt yourself and no one will be available to call 911."

- "Mom, I get nervous and anxious when the TV volume is too loud. I also worry that the apartment management may get complaints from your neighbors."

- "Dad, I worry about all those crazy people on the road who don't look out for other drivers. I will feel better if we test your response time so that you can be safer on the road."

CAREGIVER TIP:

The best and least threatening way to get your parents to talk about their wishes, needs, fears and wants as it relates to their long term care is to engage them in planning your own long term care. Tell them what you would want (*"When I get older, I want to be cared for in my home rather than in a nursing home,"* for example) and then ask them what they would want. Using this approach makes them feel like they are parenting you rather than you parenting them. It would feel like a discussion rather than you prying.

NOTES:

_____

_____

_____

_____

_____

_____

_____

_____

Engage your parents in discussions about their long term care wishes.

CHAPTER 5

When Mom and Dad Are Resistant to Care:

Here are 5 things you can do.

It can be very frustrating when your parents are having difficulty yet they refuse help. This chapter will help you to understand their position and give you five things you can do to lower their resistance and get them the help they so very much need.

Words are important. Often, they mean different things to different people. For words to be effective they must be spoken, written or shared. Without action, words are simply meaningless"

— Stella Nsong

Understanding Your Parents' Reluctance to Accept Help

When your parents refuse care, try to understand the reasons behind their resistance. Resistance to care is connected to their feelings about *help, welfare* or *loss of independence*.

Ask yourself these questions and see if you understand their position:

1. Are mom and dad concerned about cost?

2. Is a community service viewed as charity?

3. Are they afraid of having a stranger in their home?

4. Is their pride a factor?

5. Are the requirements for the use of community services overwhelming because of financial disclosure, or is the application process too involved and complicated?

Five Things You Can Do When Your Parents are Resistant to Care

1. Start small.

If your parents view government support services as "welfare," emphasize that they have paid for these services already through the taxes they have paid. If your parents are veterans, explain that they may need to receive care and prove that they qualify for the veteran pension if this is applicable to them.

Starting small is very helpful when your parents' vision, hearing, driving and personal care are involved. For example: When hearing loss is a challenge, the first change would be to install a telephone amplifier and then the next step could be a hearing assessment.

Introducing ideas slowly increases the chances for acceptance.

2. Focus on your needs with "I" statements.

If your parents insist that they are fine and they don't need any help, try focusing on your own needs rather then theirs. Here is an example of something you could say:

"I would feel better if …"

"I would feel more comfortable when I am not in town if you would let so-and-so do some errands for you on my behalf…"

"Mom, Dad, would you consider trying this service for me so I wouldn't worry so much? I really worry when you go up those steps with the laundry basket when nobody is around."

3. Suggest a trial period.

A trial period will help your parents see an end in sight. Trying something for a month is less threatening than saying, *"This is what you have to do."*

4. Employ someone familiar like a neighbor, a family friend or a fellow parishioner.

You could hire a neighbor to prepare meals or just to go over and help your parents prepare meals or clean the home, do the yard work and provide transportation.

5. Give a gift of service.

Say mom has trouble combing her hair and making her meals. Give her a gift of private care in the home. The best way to do this is for you to contact a good in-home care agency and purchase a block of care. Have the agency send a compatible caregiver dressed in street clothes and come as a homemaker with transportation. The caregiver can take her to the beauty shop and then make her some meals when they get back. When it comes time for her to have care all the time, she would be accustomed to the idea of having care.

CAREGIVER TIP:

A Medicare HMO provides skilled nursing care and rehabilitation through contracted facilities. Ensure that your loved one will be able to receive these services where he/she lives so that you can plan correctly in the event that skilled care is needed. If your loved one needs to go for rehabilitation outside of his/her continuous care community, you would want to tour a few of these facilities ahead of time so that you will be prepared should the need arise.

NOTES:

_____

_____

_____

_____

_____

_____

_____

Plan ahead for skilled nursing care and rehabilitation.

CHAPTER 6

Decision Making when Memory Loss has Started

In this chapter, we will discuss tips on how to handle decision making when your parents are not always able to participate in the decision making process.

"People will judge you by your actions, not your intentions. Sometimes actions and intentions are opposite so speak up because you may have a heart of gold but so does a hard boiled egg."

— Stella Nsong

Making the Right Decision for 99-Year-Old Company President – A True Story

Most of my clients are retired professionals. A few of them have worked until their late 90s. One memorable lady was Emma, who was still the president of her company at age 99.

Emma's memory was getting bad—and her daughter was faced with making the decision to sell her mother's business. Emma couldn't always remember the names of her employees or the face of her general manager when he would bring the payroll checks for Emma to sign. Imagine the employees not being paid because their president did not remember them. What would the general manager say to the staff when he returned with unsigned checks?

The general manager would bring the checks to Emma's home for her signatures, and my staff was always entertained during those visits. They would help Emma get dressed in her business suit and she would sit in a big chair looking exactly like the queen with each strand of hair in precisely the right place, her bright red lip stick, and her custom made clip board.

With her glasses adjusted just so over the bifocals, Emma would look over the checks and the amounts. If she did not remember the names of the employees, she would argue, and when she did not recognize the general manger she would accuse him of wanting to steal from her. When Emma was a young professional, twenty dollars was what you made a week, not an hour. These arguments happened almost every two weeks for about 2 years.

Finally one day, in her frustration with the general manager, Emma fired him—or so she thought anyway. We had written down the facts of the incident so we would have something to show her as a reminder if later she asked about him. Fortunately for us, Emma never asked about the business again… and her daughter was comfortable with making the decision to sell the business.

Prepare Yourself for the Role of Decision Maker

Only in cases of advanced Alzheimer's or a major stroke would your parents be completely unable to participate in caregiving decisions. In these kinds of cases, family members must take greater control in making and carrying out these decisions.

This is what I mean by love not being enough. Here is why.

You may experience guilt, anger, hostility and rejection from your parents when you have to make decisions for them. You may be called names and you may be called something else besides the daughter or the son. Prepare yourself for the arrows of anger and bullets of rejection. This is especially true since your parent may not be able to remember discussions or agreements that were made in the recent past.

You may find it difficult to step in and make decisions when a family member is memory impaired. It might be just as hard to step back when a relative is mentally intact and making a decision that you completely disagree with.

The decision making process can be a difficult one. Give yourself time and give your loved one patience and understanding.

Three Tips for Dealing with Your Parent's Anger and Mistrust towards You

1. Although anger may be directed at you, these feelings are really the result of the pain of the situation that they are feeling and not you. You are not the problem.

2. Because of the disease process, it is unrealistic to expect your memory-impaired parent to fully comprehend the true situation.

3. If and when you are accused of stealing their car or money, remember that to them, it feels like these things have been stolen. They may not be able to remember that they told you to sell their car, or that the doctor said they should no longer drive, or that you both agreed to move money into a care account.

Top 10 Things to Keep in Mind about Caregiving for Someone with Memory Loss

1. Dementia itself is not a disease, but is the loss of mental function in more than two of the following areas: language, judgment, memory, spatial abilities and visual abilities.

2. Dementia symptoms can be reversible or irreversible.

3. Most people with symptoms of early dementia have some form of depression. If they are truly depressed and the depression is treated, the symptoms of dementia will improve or be reversed. If your parents are experiencing symptoms of dementia, ask their doctor to test them for depression.

4. Alzheimer's disease is the most common form of dementia among older people, and age is the most common known risk factor for the disease.

5. Every day on average, 986 Americans are diagnosed with Alzheimer's disease.

6. Informal or unpaid care of the elderly has traditionally been estimated to account for 95% of all the care given to older adults.

7. Alzheimer's caregivers are twice as likely as other caregivers to provide more than 40 hours of care per week.

8. Non-spouse caregivers who are living with and providing financial support for the person with Alzheimer's disease spend an average of $261.00 a month of their own money for prescriptions drugs, clothing and other out-of-pocket expenses.

9. The average lifetime cost for each person suffering from Alzheimer's disease is $174,000. Neither Medicare nor private insurance covers the long term cost of the care that most patients need.

10. 70% of all the care provided for those with memory loss is provided in the home.

CAREGIVER TIP:

Before assets have to be spent down, make sure that you have purchased a funeral insurance plan. Preplanning and prefunding are two different things. You can preplan without prefunding but preplanning will save you lots of stress in that you can budget accordingly.

NOTES:

_____

_____

_____

_____

_____

_____

_____

_____

Preplan and budget for a funeral insurance plan.

CHAPTER 7

How to Delay or Avoid Nursing Home Placement: Seven things you can do.

Forty percent of all seniors will spend some time in a nursing home. In this chapter, we will discuss seven simple things you can do to delay or avoid nursing home placement.

"In Caregiving, nothing is simple, no decision is perfect. Let your decision making be guided by two things: risk versus benefits."

— Stella Nsong

Older Adults Get Placed in a Nursing Home for Primarily 3 Reasons:

1. A fall that causes injury and the inability to care for themselves.

2. Deconditioning that happens in the hospital or the rehab facility indicating the need for 24 hour care.

3. No willing, available or able caregiver once the need for 24 hour care has been established.

The best way to avoid or delay nursing home placement is to prevent a fall.

Here are some alarming statistics about the impact of a fall in the life of an elderly person.

▶ Every 18 seconds, an elderly person is in the emergency room because of a fall.

▶ Every 35 minutes, an older person dies because of a fall.

▶ Falls are the main cause of serious injury and accidental death in the elderly.

▶ Older adults taking four or more medications are at a higher risk for falls.

▶ The risk for falls increases with age and it is greater for women than for men.

- 67% of those who fall will fall again within six months.

- For people 65-69, one out of every 200 falls results in a hip fracture. For people 85 and older, one out of every 10 falls results in a hip fracture.

- 25% of those who fracture a hip die within six months of the injury.

- 76% of the people living in a long term care facility are there because of a fall. Most of these falls are related to problems with medications.

- Muscle weakness, loss of muscle tone, poor fitting footwear, medications for diabetes, heart conditions, blood pressure and sleep disorders can all cause falls.

- 33% of those who fall die within a year from the complications of the fall.

Seven things you can do to avoid or delay the need for nursing home placement.

1. **Get a professional home safety evaluation** and consider all the recommendations for home modifications. Safety first. If you can prevent a fall, you are almost guaranteed that a nursing home is very, very far away.

2. **Get the doctor to reevaluate the medication list.** The less medications the better. Sometimes, when there is a medical event, new medications are ordered – however, once the medical situation has been resolved, physicians often forget to stop the newer medication, or one physician may not know what the other physician ordered. Sometimes, older people take two or more medications for the same ailment ordered by two different physicians.

3. **Get all medications from the same pharmacy** so that it will be easier for drug interactions to be discovered before a crisis occurs.

4. If you realize that your loved one has suddenly become incontinent, get the doctor to **check for an infection**. Infections are a common cause of falls in the elderly population.

5. If your loved one is admitted into the hospital, do everything in your power to **help him or her to sit up each day in the chair,** and to get up and ambulate if the doctor will allow it. For every day older people lay in a hospital bed, they lose muscle tone and function. In my experience, for every day that an older adult lays in a hospital bed, it takes five to seven days to regain their pre-hospital level of functioning.

6. After three days of a hospital stay, some people will qualify for rehabilitation in a nursing home or a rehab hospital. Not everyone thrives in rehab. If you have the option, arrange for **home care and adult day care for your loved one after a hospital stay.** He/she will rehab

faster at home provided it is safe and you have a good support system. If 24-hour care is needed, and it is not in the budget, you could consider adult day care during the day and in-home care during the night. This option will reduce your cost by half.

7. **Have a long term care plan with mile stones.** By this I mean have a plan that says if mom suffers a fall, we will care for her this way. If she needs in-home care, we will pay for it that way. If dad can no longer care for mom, here will be their options. If you have a long term plan with milestones, you will be prepared for any emergency and be able to provide the best care possible for both you and your parents.

1. Get a professional home saftey evaluation

2. Get the doctor to reevaluate the medication list

3. Get all medications from the same pharmacy

4. Check for infections

5. Help your parent to sit up each day in a chair / ambulate

6. Arrange for home care and adult day care after a hospital stay

7. Have a long term care plan with mile stones

The Nightingale Story

Nightingale Home Support & Care, Inc. is one of my eldercare agencies. Located in northeast Ohio, we provide assisted living services in the home. Our services prevent older people from moving into long term care facilities. Our caregivers have three goals:

1. To relieve the caregiving stress of the family members on hand.

2. To locate, plan for, coordinate and deliver the best quality of care at the most cost effective rate available.

3. To help the older adult to find meaning and quality of life in their later years.

Based on the experiences of our clients and the notes we receive from their children, we have come to believe that our services are life changing.

You see, when an elderly person is hospitalized, things change very quickly. Something happens when you change the environment of an old person. There is confusion, agitation, forgetfulness, memory loss, falls, sudden loss of the ability to take care of their daily needs (toileting, grooming, feeding etc.) and there is also a mountain of stress. You, the caregiver, are stressing out because the hospital is saying that your loved one cannot go home unless you have 24-hour care in place.

You can't do it all by yourself. You have to work and take care of your kids, and then there is that big project at church, and you don't know if your loved one can afford that kind of help.

To make matters worse, you are worried that putting your loved one in another facility for rehab will only cause more confusion, new infections and a possible decline.

> *"Something happens when you change the environment of an old person."*

If you have ever promised not to put mom or dad in a nursing home, you have all that guilt to carry around. Meanwhile, your siblings can't imagine that you are about to spend mom and dad's money just for care.

If this sounds familiar, take heart. At Nightingale Home Support & Care, Inc., we hear this all the time and we can help. As a matter of fact, we can help you today. We can help you take your loved one home, find funds to help reduce your out-of-pocket cost (for 24-hour in-home care), nurse your loved one back to good health to the extent possible, and then we can help you keep them safe, happy and functional.

Here is what one of our clients had to say while in the hospital after fracturing a hip and a shoulder. Looking down towards the foot of the bed as the nurse adjusted the sling, the following words were said:

> *"I may not be able to walk again. Do you think my leg is shorter now? When I was 85, I fell and broke my right hip. I was gone from my home for one whole year. I was in the hospital and then rehab."*

The family of this client was fortunate to find out about Nightingale's Life Enhancement program. The Life Enhancement team was invited by the family and the doctor to join the hospital staff in providing one-on-one care in the hospital: to help do the exercises after therapy, to provide mental stimulation, to turn her every two hours (a cast and a sling made it time consuming for the hospital staff) and to do the incentive breathing exercise. In two weeks, this client was discharged to the home where the same one-on-one 24-hour care continued. In just six weeks, this client was able to walk again.

Compare six weeks of recovery after one-on-one care to one year of hospital and rehab stay. This is the power of Nightingale's Life Enhancement Program.

Call 440-942-9933 or visit www.NigtingaleHomeSupport.Com for details.

CAREGIVER TIP:

You might be eligible to receive a tax credit for up to 30% of the cost of community care services such as adult day care and in home care if you hire someone to provide care for your loved one (and make the proper social security contributions) while you work. Meet with a qualified accountant to analyze your financial options as it relates to Caregiving.

NOTES:

_____

_____

_____

_____

_____

_____

_____

_____

Analyze your financial options with an accountant.

CHAPTER 8

The 6 Steps to Making Decisions in Caregiving:

The W.E.C.A.R.E. Model

"Gold cannot be pure, and
people cannot be perfect."

— Chinese Proverb

The W.E.C.A.R.E. Model: The Wheel to Drive Your Caring Situation

W.E.C.A.R.E. is a decision making model that I have developed over the last two decades. It stands for

<u>W</u>elcome professional services

<u>E</u>ngage the care recipient

<u>C</u>reate care options

<u>A</u>ct on an option

<u>R</u>eassess the situation

<u>E</u>nhance independence

I call it W.E.C.A.R.E. because the most effective care plans are those that involve the caregiver, the care recipient, their wishes, their strengths and their need to feel alive and to enjoy more life out of days than days out of life. Many families have used this system in different degrees for different situations. It has one goal: To give the best care possible in the situation that you find yourself.

Imagine the caregiver at the center of a wheel. Around the CARE wheel should be:

1. Welcome professional services to give you an objective picture of the situation.

2. Engage the care recipient and discover their wishes.

3. Create realistic care options around the care recipient's wishes.

4. Act on an option.

5. Reassess the situation and the outcomes of the care option that you have acted upon.

6. Enhance independence to the extent possible.

The CARE Wheel

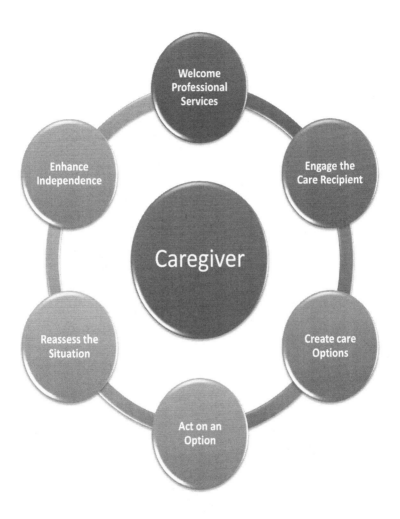

Three Tips for Making Successful Decisions in Caregiving

1. Allow your parents to take some risk.

   It is natural to want to overprotect your parent especially when he or she is getting frail. However, that is usually the last thing an older person wants or needs. Too much protection can undermine your parent's self-esteem. The goal is to try for a balance in caring. Allow your parents to continue to carry out functions that they can still do even if with difficulty. If you take everything away, that may cause resistance, depression and dependence.

2. Safety should be first, not everything.

   Safety is important but it is not the only thing. It is just as important to focus on the remaining abilities of your parents, as it is to focus on the limitations. You want to avoid forcing your values on your parents. What you think is best may not always be true. Very often, adult children are concerned with the parent's "quantity of life" but the parent is concerned with "quality of life."

3. Avoid promises. You may not be able to live up to them.

   Try not to make promises like:

   "I will never put you in a nursing home."

   "You can always live with us."

   "You can always stay in your home."

   "I will quit my job and take care of you if you need me to."

What may seem like the best solution today may not be the same ten years from now when your own health or that of your parent's has changed. Unfulfilled promises often result in guilt, anger, mistrust and disappointment.

Beware of the "Shoulds"

Also, watch out for the "shoulds" in caregiving. These usually come from guilt. If your parent's health deteriorates, you may find yourself with "shoulds" like these:

- A caring daughter should invite her parents to move in with her.

- A good son should not allow his mother to live alone.

- A responsible child should quit her job to care for her parents.

"Shoulds" may come from guilt within you, from other family members, from outside the family, from your parent's friends or from people who should not even matter like the mail carrier or the neighbor's housekeeper. It's important not to let the guilt of "shoulds" guide your decisions.

Guilt can create very destructive outcomes: end a career, destroy a marriage, destroy mental health, destroy physical health or even sacrifice healthy relationships. Guilt can reduce objectivity, reduce your ability to decide on what is best for you, your parents and your family.

If a promise you are unable to keep is the source of "shoulds" guilt, anger and frustrations, look back at the conditions under which you made those promises and compare them with the situation today. Most likely, the conditions are very different. Comparing *what is* with *what was* may help to give you clarity and an objective look at the current situation. That might make it easier for you to let go of a promise that is now completely unrealistic to keep. Forgive yourself and focus on the here and the now.

CAREGIVER TIP:

Ask your parent's opinion as to who should handle the money and who should be in charge of their health care. Most parents would choose based on how their children were in childhood and they would be less resentful when tough decisions have to be made. Ask these questions now and document the answers somewhere, especially if advanced directives have not been executed. It will become useful amongst the family members who are involved in the Caregiving.

NOTES:

_____

_____

_____

_____

_____

_____

_____

_____

Ask your parents who should handle the money and be in charge of their health care.

CHAPTER 9

Guides to Hiring the Right Caregiving Help

This chapter provides three guides that will help you find the best in-home medical and non-medical agency or assisted living community for your given situation:

- How to Hire a Caregiver Privately
- How to Choose a Home Care Provider
- How to Choose an Assisted Living Facility

"It is not only what we do, but also what we do not do for which we are accountable."

— Moliere

Private Aide Sues her Wealthy Employer

In 2004, I had a client that every aide would want to have. A retired doctor, Tom was very particular about things such as his food and his office at home. Otherwise, Tom was very funny, very intelligent, and hated Medicare rules and regulations when it came to being home bound.

The aides enjoyed caring for Tom because he loved to travel, loved good food and entertainment, and he was cantankerous—all at the same time. My staff traveled with him all over the country by airplane and in his motor home. He had a few mobility problems but nothing stopped him. Tom had a great lifestyle but as time went on, frugality replaced good judgment. After about a year of very good and comprehensive care from our agency, he was feeling better and he thought that he could manage his own care.

One day, Tom decided he would cut back from round-the-clock care through our agency to night care and some daytime care with a private aide. This was the way he was going to reduce his cost of care. He had enough funds to pay for round-the-clock care until the age of one hundred and five if he could live that long. Cutting the care was not a financial necessity. It was a need to feel like he had control over his care and his life.

Tom hired a very mature private caregiver to provide care for him eight hours a day, five days a week from 8 a.m. to 4 p.m. The agency staff would provide care from 7 p.m. to 7 a.m. and the rest of the time, he thought he could manage on his own. I gave Tom a list of things to consider as he offered the new caregiver this private care position. He did not take my recommendations at the time.

Things went well for about a week and a half. One day, the private caregiver was doing laundry and slipped on a rug and injured her knee and her back. The emergency room filed a worker's compensation claim because the caregiver said that she got injured at work. There was no signed contract between my wealthy client and the caregiver… and so Tom was sued for loss of income, injury, pain and suffering and partial disability. Her lawyers argued that my client was the employer because he told her when to come to work and what to do. The cost of the lawsuit was hundreds of times more than the few dollars he saved by hiring the caregiver privately.

How to Hire a Caregiver Privately

The choice to stay at home almost always requires some type of assistance, help and service from others. For most older adults, staying at home and having care brought into the home is the most preferred form of long term care. It is important to educate yourself especially if you choose to hire a caregiver privately.

> *"Use this guide to protect your family and to shield your parents from federal, state and local taxation and labor requirements."*

Some families choose to hire privately, rather than to go through a home health care agency because of cost and flexibility of scheduling.

Sometimes it's because of the need for the older adult to feel as if he/she has an "assistant" instead of a caregiver. An older adult will often be more receptive to an "assistant" than to a "caregiver." This is a common occurrence for those retired executives and professionals who are struggling with the loss of their independence.

It is important to note that when you hire a caregiver privately, he/she does not have to be licensed by the state or be Medicare approved. You will need to do the investigation of the individual to be sure that he/she is honest, reliable and capable of performing the services that you want and need. A home care agency makes sure that their staff will show up if the person you hired is ill or takes a vacation. If you hire privately, you will be without that person or that back up.

Whatever your situation may be, if you choose to hire a caregiver privately—and thus choose to perform the functions of "The Employer"— use this guide to protect your family and to shield your parents from federal, state and local taxation and labor requirements.

Checklist to Ensure that You Hire an Honest, Reliable and Resourceful Caregiver

1. Do an FBI check if the person has lived outside of your state in the last five years.

2. Check the national registry for certified home health aides if the person is certified as a home health aide.

3. Have a written contract with the caregiver stating who is responsible for federal, state and local unemployment and worker's compensation taxes.

4. Check if the caregiver has car insurance.

5. Check if the caregiver has a clean driving record.

6. Make sure the caregiver is free of communicable disease and has no physical limitations.

7. Have a system for handling credit cards, money and cash in the home.

8. Make sure your parent's vital information is in a secured location.

9. Make sure your parent's valuables are in a locked and secured location.

10. Have a system to serve as backup care in case your private caregiver is sick or on vacation.

How to Choose a Home Care Provider

What to look for when hiring nursing care at home	Nightingale Home Support & Care Inc. 866-933-6442	Another Agency	Another Agency
Payment plans and discounts based on level of care	☑	☐	☐
Service available immediately - as soon as you call on us	☑	☐	☐
TELL US YOUR STORY AND WE WILL CREATE A CARE PLAN JUST FOR YOU	☑	☐	☐
Client and family collaboration in developing the plan of care	☑	☐	☐
Free evaluation and cost analysis of other care options	☑	☐	☐
Written statements explaining services, cost, payment schedules, insurance and grants available	☑	☐	☐
Caregivers are screened, insured/bonded and are selected for their maturity, skill and experience	☑	☐	☐
Transportation, support groups, family education and access to other caregiving resources	☑	☐	☐
Registered Nurse on call 24 hours a day, 7 days a week	☑	☐	☐
Flexible, intermittent and around-the-clock services available immediately	☑	☐	☐
Strict documentation and maintenance of patient rights and confidentiality	☑	☐	☐
Strict RN supervision of all caregivers	☑	☐	☐
Accreditation and certificate of good business standing	☑	☐	☐

How to Choose an Assisted Living Facility

Assisted living is a confusing care alternative for many people. I have met several families who did not understand what the level of care should be in an assisted living facility, or the kinds of services offered. They did not understand how to help their loved one make the transition until after their loved one had moved in and discovered that it was completely different from what their expectations were.

Assisted living can be a very good care option for the older adult who wants to be social, active and as functional as possible. These kinds of people can thrive in assisted living. For those who do not want to go to assisted living but have no other good option at the time, consider using assisted living as a short term option following the decision making model and the CARE wheel on pages 55 and 56.

The Levels of Care in Assisted Living Facilities

Generally, assisted living services are structured on three levels of care. Four factors are used to measure the level of care:

1. Cognitive impairment

2. Ability to manage medications

3. Need for care from a licensed nurse on the facility staff

4. Level of physical impairment requiring hands-on care with activities of daily living.

The higher the level of care, the more costly the services will be.

A Guide to Determine the Level of Care Provided
in Some Assisted Living Facilities

CATEGORY	LEVEL 1	LEVEL 2	LEVEL 3
Cognitive Impairments	Occasional prompts	Daily cuing and prompts	Ongoing cuing, prompts, and redirection
Medication Administration	Independent with medications (Requires no staff involvement)	Supervision with medication management (Staff involvement with procurement, storage and reminders)	Medication administration by qualified staff
Nursing	No individualized scheduled, hands-on care provided by a licensed nurse, assisted living staff	Weekly and/or monthly individualized, hands-on care provided by a licensed nurse	Daily nursing care due to an unstable medical condition or intermittent skilled nursing care provided by the facility
Physical Impairments indicating a need for hands-on assistance with ADL's	Individuals who require up to 2.75 hours of service per day	Individuals who require more than 2.75 hours and less than 3.5 hours of service per day	Individuals who require more than 3.5 hours of service per day

Note: The category with the highest level assignment determines the level that will be assigned. Example: If a client meets Level 2 for Cognitive Impairments and Level 3 for Medication Administration, Level 3 will be the assignment.

Assisted Living to Independent Living…

A success story at the Woodlands at Eastland
Columbus Ohio 43232 (614) 866-2080

I am the eldercare consultant of the Woodlands at Eastland, an independent and assisted living community on the east side of Columbus, Ohio. I am a big advocate for aging in place for in-home care but sometimes, in-home care is not possible. Sometimes, assisted living is the best option.

Using the WECARE model, the Woodlands at Eastland has many success stories. The key is striving for independence and involving the care recipient and the family caregiver. Our youngest residents are in their 50s and our oldest residents are just a little over 100 years old… and I am proud to say, with the right music and a little help, most of them can get up and dance. We are a community of active retirees.

Here is the story of one of our residents.

After a diagnosis of lung cancer, Jack was sent to a rehabilitation center where he spent three months receiving therapy. He "plateaued" as a physical therapist would say, and it was time for discharge. He was too sick to go home but not sick enough to be hospitalized and he refused to wait and die in a nursing home. According to him, a nursing home is a "human warehouse."

Jack has no children and had lost his wife several years ago to a long battle with cancer. He has a distant relative, Steve, who stepped up to serve as power of attorney and caregiver. Steve had a friend whose brother lived at the Woodlands. Steve knows how well the residents at the Woodlands thrive so he approached me for some advice.

We used the WECARE model and got Jack into assisted living. On admission, Jack had oxygen, he was wheelchair bound from generalized weakness, he needed insulin almost four times a day, and he was anxious, depressed and very impatient.

We put Jack on our wellness program and within one year, we were able to discharge Jack to the independent living section of the facility.

Jack is ambulatory, needs no oxygen, no insulin, he does his own laundry, he goes out with friends who come and pick him up for outings two to three times a week, he participates in activities, and yes, he actually has a girlfriend now. They are both in their eighties and enjoying every bit of their retirement.

> **W.E.C.A.R.E. Model**
>
> **W**elcome professional services
>
> **E**ngage the care recipient
>
> **C**reate care options
>
> **A**ct on an option
>
> **R**eassess the situation
>
> **E**nhance independence

Everybody can't be this successful in assisted living; but if you must use this option, then use the guide on the next page to locate the best possible assisted living facility for your loved one.

Guide to Choosing an Assisted Living Facility

What to look for when selecting an Assisted Living Facility		
	Woodlands at Eastland Columbus, Ohio 43232 (614) 866-2080	Another Facility
Free wellness program to prevent de-conditioning and enhance recovery.	✓	
Weekly phone call to the families to provide an update and support.	✓	
Bimonthly family caregiver support program.	✓	
Biweekly Circle of Gratitude open to all residents and family members.	✓	
One set monthly cost regardless of the level of care.	✓	
Written statement explaining services, cost, payments and insurance.	✓	
You have a choice about the level of care you desire.	✓	
Occupancy available today.	✓	
Resident and family participation in developing and enhancing the plan of care.	✓	
RN on call 24 hours a day, 7 days a week. RN supervisor for all caregivers.	✓	
Social and recreational programs available.	✓	
Licensed driver and local transportation available every day. Come see our clean bus.	✓	
State and Federal background checks on all employees, including fingerprinting and drug screen.	✓	
Specially trained Life Enhancement Caregivers for post surgery, chronic diseases and Alzheimer's care.	✓	
Elder care consultant and long term care planner on site.	✓	
VA Benefits consultant on site.	✓	
Extra special care and higher security care for those challenged by memory loss and sundowners syndrome.	✓	
Medicare skilled services available.	✓	
One level ranch style suites with screened patio overlooking oriental gardens.	✓	

CAREGIVER TIP:

It is prudent to hire providers who are insured and bonded, but bear in mind that a bond would only pay for a claim if the person involved is convicted. Keep valuables in a safe place and do not disclose financial information with your direct care providers even if the agency they represent is insured and bonded. Insurance and bonding is not 100% protection.

NOTES:

_____

_____

_____

_____

_____

_____

_____

_____

_____

Take measures to protect your valuables and financial information in your caregiving setting.

CHAPTER 10

Long Term Care Planning Survey:
Begin putting your long term care plan together

In this chapter, you will discover what your parent's care preferences
are, what kind of professional help you might need along the way, and
what kind of documents and caregiving tools you will need to be an
informed caregiver. Based on your situation, you might actually end up
with your own very care plan.

"Sometimes, doing nothing is actually doing something. You don't have to take action blindly…but act you must if anything is to ever be accomplished."

Stella Nsong

Where to Begin Your Long Term Care Plan

The long term care plan is the plan for how and where your parents will hopefully age in place.

The first thing to do is to conduct the care planning survey on the following pages. This will help you to determine

- your parent's preferences for care;

- the areas for which you need to gather more information;

- which professionals you need to contact to help you design the long term plan of care for your parents.

Long Term Care Planning Survey

In each blank, place #1 to #5 with #1 being the highest preference. Determining care preferences will allow you to decide whether your parents want to remain in the home, go to a retirement community like an assisted living facility, or make other living arrangements. The information in the care plan survey will be coming from your parents and not from you so they will be providing these answers to you to the best of their abilities.

Preferences for future care providers. (Put in each blank, #1 to #5, #1 is highest preference).

_____ A family member will provide care, with help from other family or professionals.

_____ A friend will provide care, possibly with help from professionals.

_____ A home health agency or personal care agency will provide care.

_____ Care will be provided by the staff of an assisted living facility.

_____ Care will be provided by the staff of a nursing home.

Preferences for the future care setting in which you want your own long-term care to take place. (Put in each blank, preferences from #1 to #5, #1 being highest preference).

_____ Remain in your own home as long as possible.

_____ Live with a family member or friend as long as possible.

_____ Live in a retirement community or independent living complex as long as possible.

_____ Live in a congregate care or assisted living facility.

_____ Live in a nursing home.

Preferences for your spouse's future care providers. (Put in each blank, preferences from #1 to #5, #1 being highest preference.

_____ A family member will provide care, with help from other family or professionals.

_____ A friend will provide care, possibly with help from professionals.

_____ A home health agency or personal care agency will provide care.

_____ Care will be provided by the staff of an assisted living facility.

_____ Care will be provided by the staff of a nursing home.

Preferences for the future care setting in which spouse wants long term care to take place. (Put in each blank, preferences from #1 to #5, #1 being highest preference.

_____ Remain in your own home as long as possible.

_____ Live with a family member or friend as long as possible.

_____ Live in a retirement community or independent living complex as long as possible.

_____ Live in a congregate care or assisted living facility.

_____ Live in a nursing home.

Does the care recipient have someone who can act as a Care Coordinator? This could be a family member, friend or a paid professional.

_____ Yes   _____ No

If Yes, what is the relationship of that person to you? _____

If No, have you considered the services of a Professional Care Manager? _____ Yes _____ No

Name of Care Coordinator: _____

Contact information for Care Coordinator: _____

The Care Coordinator will work with the current or future potential caregiver.

Will the caregiver be a family member? _____ Yes   _____ No

Will the caregiver be a professional service provider? _____ Yes   _____ No

Name of Caregiver: _____

Address of Caregiver: _____

Phone Number of Caregiver: _____

Does care recipient and/or spouse have any of the following documents?

_____ Will?   _____ For Spouse?   Date of last review: _____

_____ Living Will?   _____ For Spouse?

Does the care recipient have any of the following documents for himself/herself?

(Check those that are applicable)

_____ General Power of Attorney

_____ Durable Power of Attorney

_____ Medical Power of Attorney

Does the spouse (if it pertains) have any of the following documents for himself/herself? (Check those that are applicable.)

_____ General Power of Attorney

_____ Durable Power of Attorney

_____ Medical Power of Attorney

Does anyone in the care recipient household have any of the following types of trusts?

_____ Family or Living Trust   Date of last review: _____

_____ Charitable Remainder Trust   Date of last review: _____

_____ Generation Skipping Trust   Date of last review: _____

_____ Other Trusts   Date of last review: _____

Is there a family limited partnership? _____ Yes   _____ No

Do you need advice with strategies to lessen the financial burden of Medicaid? ___ Yes ___ No
Medicaid rules are different from state to state and they change frequently—so if you answer Yes to this question, consider the services and advice of a certified eldercare attorney or an estate planning attorney.

Does the care recipient or family have a need requiring the advice of an elder law attorney or estate planning attorney? _____ Yes   _____ No

Does the care recipient have private insurance to pay for the cost of care? _____ Yes _____ No

Are there any other financial arrangements to pay the cost of care? _____ Yes _____ No

Have you made a list of the following accounts or insurance policies for the Personal Care Coordinator?

_____ Bank accounts, checking, savings, safe deposit box

_____ Tax deferred savings accounts

_____ Retirement funds such as pension, etc.

_____ Annuities and trusts

_____ Life insurance policies

_____ Health insurance policies

_____ Long term care insurance policies

_____ Medicare Insurance information

_____ Other accounts for policies

_____

_____

_____

_____

Real estate assets owned by the care recipient or spouse/child living in the home

_____ Personal Residence

_____ Second Residence, cabin, rental, etc.

_____ Investment Property

_____ Business

Do you need advice about Long Term Care Insurance? _____ Yes _____ No

Do you need help with Medicare Insurance, advantage plans? _____ Yes _____ No

Do you need advice from a retirement planner? _____ Yes _____ No

Do you need a Senior Real Estate Specialist to consult with selling real property?

_____ Yes _____ No

Are you aware of community services in your area?

_____ Senior Centers

_____ Area Agencies on Aging

_____ Church and community aging support groups

If the care recipient has traditional Medicare, an Advantage Plan or a prescription drug plan, do you know the benefits:

_____ Inpatient Hospital

_____ Nursing Home

_____ Home Health Care

_____ Hospice

_____ Outpatient medical care

_____ Drug benefits

If the care recipient is a war veteran or the surviving widow of a veteran, he or she might receive additional income to help pay for a nursing home, assisted living, or home care.

Do you understand the VA qualifications? _____ Yes _____ No

Do you know how to apply for benefits? _____ Yes _____ No

Do you need more information on VA benefits: _____ Yes _____ No

Do you need help understanding Medicare and Medicaid Services? _____ Yes _____ No

Did you serve at least ninety (90) days on active duty during a period of war, or are you the surviving spouse of such a Veteran? _____ Yes _____ No

Your Next Steps – Creating a Long Term Care Plan

Once you have completed the survey, the next step would be to get a care agreement in place with your parents and all those who will be involved in their care.

Follow these steps and before you know it, you will have everything under control.

1. Gather any missing information as reflected on the results of your survey.

   Here are some examples:

   If one parent tells you that there is a will but you can't find the will, go through their phone book and find their attorney and contact him or her to get a copy of the will. What if your dad served in the military and you can't find his discharge paper? Look for the steel box in the closet, the office in the house, the basement or the attic. If that fails, go to the Veterans Administration website and request a copy. You could also get assistance in obtaining another copy through your local veteran service officer.

2. If you need professionals to help you design the long term care plan, this is the time to contact them. The best place to find quick and affordable help is through the National Care Planning Council. That website is www.longtermcarelink.net. Through this website, you will be able to reach professionals in your area who specialize in the kind of help that you will need.

   Here is an example.

   If your parents do not have a signed and notarized power of attorney or a living will, you will need the services of an estate planning attorney or an eldercare attorney. Do not wait until memory loss starts. Everyone should have a signed and notarized power of attorney. If memory loss has started, you will not be able to do a power of attorney document. You will need to pursue guardianship, which can be a very time consuming and expensive process.

3. With the help of the professionals and your parents, develop options.

4. Pick an option and set a trial period and then execute that option.

5. Reassess the situation.

6. Adjust the care options as needed and strive to enhance your parents' independence. Remember to focus on **more life out of days** than **days out of life**. Measure their "quantity of life" versus "length of life" by their standards, not yours. For older adults, each day is quantified into hours and minutes of experiencing life. Do what you can to enable them to feel alive each day and enjoy the small yet important things that they want to do.

CAREGIVER TIP:

As you spend down, make sure that you have purchased a funeral insurance plan and all durable medical equipment (lift chairs, stand up lifts, stair lift, etc.) that is needed to make Caregiving safer and easier.

NOTES:

_____

_____

_____

_____

_____

_____

_____

_____

Purchase funeral insurance and medical equipment with spend down.

A Final Word

It is my hope that this little book has helped you to find possible solutions to your Caregiving situation. As you have gone through this book, I hope that each chapter has helped you to feel more and more in control of your situation, and that through these tips and actions steps, you will be able to design your own successful CARE wheel.

I hope that these stories will help you keep things in perspective and that some of the quotes have brought a smile to your face—even when all you want to do is cry and wish that your parents had told you all the things that you are now having to discover by force. Whatever your situation is, give yourself credit for being a caregiver, because not everyone is cut out to be one.

It takes a special person to be a caregiver. No matter how hard you try, your loved one may criticize you and blame you, even when you cannot figure out why, even when you know nothing about what's causing their anger, fear or resentment. You will get blamed for doing what you were asked to do. Sometimes your loved one will listen to complete strangers instead of you.

Take one day at a time and remember that in Caregiving, LOVE IS NOT ENOUGH. Being the best caregiver means taking care of you so that you can take care of Caregiving. Taking care of you means being stable and balanced like a 3-legged stool: It takes you, the eldercare professionals and the government/community long term care programs.

Sometimes, the strongest thing you can do is to ask for help. Help is just a phone call or click away!

About the Author

Stella Nsong, RN, CMC, CDP, LTCP

Care Manager Certified
Certified Dementia Practitioner
Long Term Care Planner

Stella Nsong has been a nurse for more than twenty years and has worked in almost every branch of health care. Over 15 years ago, Stella became a business owner, and has owned, created, started, turned around, licensed and managed private duty home care agencies, Medicare certified agencies, Medicaid certified agencies, medical adult day care centers, medical alert system companies, home medical supply companies and assisted living facilities.

Stella currently serves as the State Director of the Ohio Elder Care Planning Council, as well as the chair person for the Aging Committee of ACHIEVE in Lake County, Ohio. ACHIEVE stands for Action Communities in Health Innovation and EnVironmental Change.

Stella is a widely renowned public speaker on the topics of Elder Care and Caregiving. She has previously authored 3 other books on eldercare and is a coauthor for the Gratitude Project for 2013. Stella also is the writer and editor of the Elder Care Cliff Report, a publication of the CAREgiving Institute of Ohio.

Your purchase of this book will go to support the work of the Caring 4 Caregiver's program, a service of the CAREgiving Institute. The CAREgiving Institute is a 501(c)(3) organization whose mission is to transform America's Caregiving Crisis by providing Resources and Options for Today's and Tomorrow's Elderly.

Stella Nsong is an active member of the following professional organizations:

National Association of Professional Geriatric Care Managers
National Academy of Certified Care Managers
National Care Planning Council
Ohio Care Planning Council
National Council of Certified Dementia Practitioners

Follow Stella

http://www.StellaNsong.com/